The

MEDICARE CODE

Unlocking the Secrets To Healthcare After 65

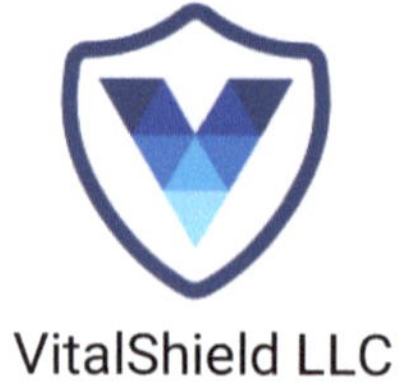

VitalShield LLC

Table of Contents

Introduction to The Medicare Code

Welcome to *The Medicare Code*. As someone born and raised in Minnesota, I've seen firsthand how the world of Medicare can vary from state to state and by zip code—it needs to be more clear!

Minnesota, for instance, has unique plans for Medicare supplements that differ from the standard Plan G found in most states - you'll learn more about supplements in this book.. Instead of the typical Plan G, we have options that, while similar, go by different names and offer unique benefits tailored to our residents. It can get confusing - especially if you're moving to another state that isn't standard.

A vivid memory about being from Minnesota comes to mind: I was in a fishing contest in Mexico with a friend when I overheard someone from Texas say, "Hey, there's those boys from Minnesota – listen to them talk!" I wanted to say isn't that a laugh - listen to you! It was the first time I realized our accents and perhaps even our perspectives were distinct. It finally dawned on me why people would ask me where I was from! I thought they were being friendly. Ha! I hope my Minnesota style will not only demystify Medicare's complexities but also resonate with readers nationwide, making you feel understood and valued. There are a few states without traditional Medicare. Minnesota, Massachusetts, and Wisconsin. So, that can add to the confusion. They have unique benefits and plans.

If you, like me, always believed that turning 65 meant health insurance would become a non-issue thanks to Medicare, prepare for a revelation. You're in for a significant surprise. This book is for you!

Having worked in the insurance business for almost 20 years, I've navigated various lines of insurance successfully. Yet, Medicare was uncharted territory for me until recently. I didn't know what I didn't know! I bet you don't either.

As I approach that crucial age – even though it feels like I was only 21 yesterday – I'm not just an insurance agent and the owner of VitalShield Insurance Services branching out into a new field; I'm also a prospective beneficiary seeking guidance through the often confusing Medicare landscape.

I remember one agent remarking that the more he studied Medicare, the more confused he became, and the more it felt like he knew nothing about it! I aim to make it easier and spare you from that ordeal. To become a Medicare expert, I attended carrier meetings, loads of conferences, and seminars, obtained my certifications, took classes, discussed plans and options to help others, read almost every book I could find, and dug deep to achieve competence.

I wrote this book from two perspectives: that of a seasoned insurance professional and that of someone who is beginning to consider health insurance and Medicare seriously as retirement approaches. Many of you probably share these feelings. It's for those of us who see 65 on the horizon, not quite there but aware it's coming, people turning 65—it's estimated over 11,000 people a day are turning 65. It's for anyone else striving to demystify Medicare.

Initially, approaching Medicare felt like opening a puzzle box without the picture on the cover. Terms like "Medigap," "Part B," and "Advantage Plans" seemed like pieces of an unsolvable puzzle. However, over the last couple of years, as I delved deeper, the picture began to take shape. My journey into understanding Medicare wasn't just about professional growth; it became a personal quest to understand what awaits me and millions of others in this age group. There is no best-choice plan - everyone's needs and options are unique.

This book attempts to peel back the layers of Medicare, moving beyond the basic overviews and getting to the core of what it means for those approaching 65. Through my journey, I've gathered insights, experiences, and knowledge I wish to share with you.

Let's navigate this journey together, uncover the intricacies of Medicare, and ensure you're well-prepared for what lies ahead. Welcome to *The Medicare Code*. Let's get to Cracking.

Chapter 1
Cracking the Medicare Part A Code

Hey there, it's Tim Peddycoart with VitalShield Insurance, and today we are delving deep into the world of Medicare. First up, Medicare Part A. Also known as "Hospital Insurance." It's probably best to buckle up as it's going to be a wild ride. No worries - I'll get you there!

Unveiling Part A Coverage:

First things first: what is the situation with part A of Medicare? You'll receive this automatically when you start collecting social security.

Consider it your lucky charm for receiving inpatient care. We're talking about stays in hospitals, assisted living centers, and even hospice services.

Let's dissect it:

1. Hospital Care: General hospital services, food, and your semi-private room are covered by part A. Furthermore, it takes effect for inpatient treatment centers and critical access to hospitals.

2. Care at expert Nursing Facilities (SNF's): should you require expert.

3. Hospice Care: This is where Part A really shines when you or a loved on is facing a terminal disease. It covers emotional support, symptom management, and pain treatment.

4. Home Health care: When you're recovering at home, Part A covers treatment, some medical supplies, and part-time nursing care that is medically needed.

The Part A Club: Who gets in?

Let's now discuss eligibility. You're probably in if you're 65 years of age or older and you or your spouse have worked for and paid in for at least ten years, sacrificing toiling, blood, sweat, and tears, well taxes - at least. However, you can also become a member if you have end-stage renal disease (ESRD) or certain disabilities and are under 65.

The Financial Conversation:

 Now for the bit nobody enjoys the money part. Some people may not need to pay a monthly premium for Part A, while others may.

But there's still more! Deductibles and coinsurance are also introduced to the parties in Part A, particularly. If your hospital stay lasts longer than a predetermined number of days as well. You're stuck with the bill once you've used those up.

The bottom line is that Medicare Part A functions as a kind of backstage pass for inpatient care. It's helpful when needed, but you must understand it's details, like coinsurance, deductibles, and premiums. As we proceed, we'll cover those specifics, so stay tuned.

We're just getting started, so get ready. Medicare is like an onion with many layers, but together we'll peel them off and make sure you know enough to choose the best healthcare. Stay tuned for Chapter 2, we'll be talking Medicare Part B with the same zeal.

Chapter 2
Decoding The Medicare Mysteries of Part B

Forging ahead into the wonderful world of Medicare. We're going to crack open the treasure chest known as Medicare Part B. So put your hat on and let's get going!

Part B: Your Health Partner:

Medicare part B, sometimes referred to as "medical insurance," is what you should use when you need necessary medical services. Consider medical appointments, outpatient treatment, health maintenance, and more. It all comes down to being well and identifying problems before they become severe headaches.

What's included in Part B Coverage:

1. Doctor's Services: Part B covers routine examinations, consultations, and specialized visits.

2. Outpatient Care: Part B covers the costs of any lab work or procedures you do in outpatient type of settings. Providing convenience and peace of mind.

3. Preventive Services: Part B promotes proactively taking charge of your health. Obtain screenings, vaccinations, and preventative care without going over budget.

4. Durable Medical Equipment (DME): Do you require a home hospital bed, wheelchair, or oxygen? Part B covers those things.

Who gets in this Part B Club:

Ok, let's talk about eligibility. If you're already in the Part A club, You're probably in the Part B too. However, pay attention here: Part B comes with a monthly premium. The amount can vary depending on your income, so it is best to be prepared.

Annual Deductibles and Coinsurance:

Like any good insurance plan, Part B has its share of costs. You'll have an annual deductible to meet before it kicks in, and after that, you typically pay 20% of the Medicare-approved amount for most services. It's not a set fee, so the cost depends on the service.

Skipping past Part B because there is a cost involved could be a costly mistake. Trying to save some cash now can lead to significant penalties later. So don't let it slide. You want to pay attention and don't assume or take things for granted.

There could be a late enrollment penalty. It's a 10% increase for every 12-month period. It's not just a one-time penalty. It sticks with you as long as you have part B. If you skip it for 3 years that's an extra 30% you'll pay.

Part B and Preventive Care:

Part B: it's all about prevention. Regular check-ups, screenings, and vaccines are your best defense against more significant health issues down the road. Think of it as an investment in your long-term well-being.

Staying informed is Key:

 Navigating Medicare Part B can feel like deciphering a secret code. But here's the secret: knowledge is power. The more you understand how it works, the better you can make it work.

In our next chapter, we'll dive into the exciting world of Medicare Advantage (Part C). It's all about choices and finding the plan that suits your needs – everyone seems to have an opinion. It's best to form your own and not listen to Uncle Cheapskate Charlie or Nervous Nancy next door who heard something. So, keep that curiosity alive, and we'll see you in the next chapter!

Chapter 3
Unlocking the Potential of Medicare Advantage
(Part C)

More Medicare Wisdom! In this Chapter, we'll explore Medicare Advantage, or Part C. Prepare yourself for an entirely new range of choices and opportunities.

Medicare Advantage: A Comprehensive Approach or an "All in One" option:

Medicare Advantage plans are comparable to the medical equivalent of Swiss Army Knives. They include benefits of Parts A and B while often adding extras like prescription drug coverage, vision, dental and more! It's one stop shopping for your health needs. Many love it for the ease and extras. Some don't care for them depending on their area network along with health and lifestyle consideration.

Medicare Advantage plans seem to work best for areas that have a lot of networks. In remote areas with fewer option it can be a challenge. We'll explore more about the Medicare Advantage Plans as we go. Your choice will become clear.

Medicare Advantage Plan Types:

1. Health Maintenance Organization (HMO): Plans under an HMO usually entail selecting a primary care physician (PCP) and obtaining referrals to see a specialist. They frequently include a network of medical professionals.

2. PPO (Preferred Provider Organization): PPO policies offer increased adaptability. You can see any doctor, specialist, or healthcare provider, but it will cost less if you stay in the network.

3. Private Fee For Service (PFFS): With PFFS plans, you can see any Medicare-approved provider who agrees to accept the plans terms. Keep in mind that not all healthcare providers may accept PFFS plans.

4. Special needs Plans (SNPs): Are designed for individuals with specific health conditions or are dual-eligible for Medicare and Medicaid.

Prescription Drug Coverage (Part D):

Many Medicare Advantage Plans include prescription drug coverage (Part D). This means you can get your medications with one plan, making managing your prescriptions more convenient.

Extra Benefits and perks:

Part C plans often spice up the deal with additional benefits like dental, vision, hearing, and even gym memberships. It's like having healthcare with VIP access. Many members belong to many gyms and take join friends in different activities.

Enrollment and Costs:

To join a Medicare Advantage Plan, you must have both Medicare Parts A and B. Plus you'll continue to pay your Part B premium, along with any additional premium the plan may charge. Costs can vary, so be sure to compare plans in your area.

Don't be afraid to have a local agent help you. It won't cost you any more to get some guidance or recommendations. The insurance companies pay them.

Yearly changes and Open Enrollment:

It's essential to keep an eye on your Medicare Advantage Plan. The coverage, costs, and benefits can change from year to year. The annua; Enrollment Period (AEP) is your chance to review and make changes if necessary. It usually runs from October 15th to December 7th each year.

Making the Right Choice:

Selecting the Right Medicare Advantage Plan requires some research and consideration. You'll want to access your healthcare needs, preferred providers, and budget to find the plan that aligns best with your lifestyle.

Some think of Medicare supplement plans as a pay now for peace of mind later and of Medicare advantage plans as pay when you use them.

If you put some money aside just in case, there are some good advantage plans and networks in your zip code, you're healthy and rarely go to the doctor then these plans could be awesome.

I'd recommend finding a good agent who represents many plans then comparing all the columns and make a choice from there. It can be easier to see them all compared and weigh each one. Using an experienced agent – contrary to what you might be thinking - won't cost you anything but will make it much easier as they should be on top of any changes and know which plans would work well in your area and for needs.

In the next chapter, we'll delve into the world of Medicare Part D – the prescription drug coverage that can save you a load of money on your prescriptions. So, stay tuned and keep exploring your Medicare options!

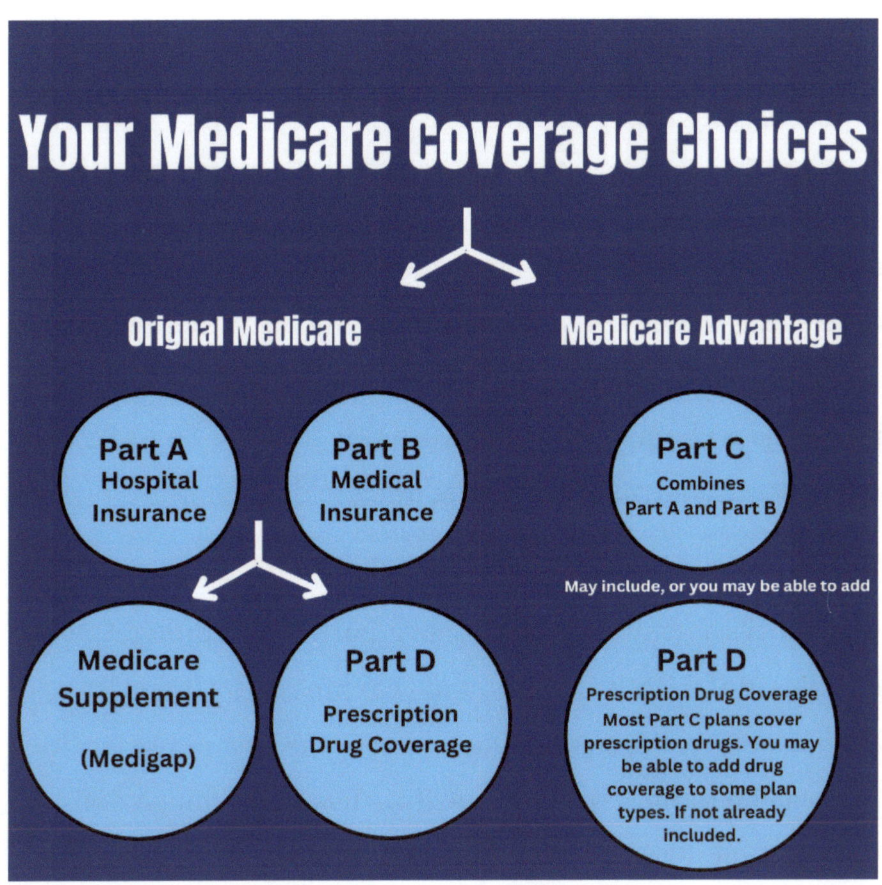

Your Medicare Coverage Choices
Orignal Medicare
Medicare Advantage
Part A
Hospital
Insurance
Part B
Medical
Insurance
Part C
Combines
Part A and Part B
May include, or you may be able to add
Medicare
Supplement
(Medigap)
Part D
Prescription
Drug Coverage
Part D
Prescription Drug Coverage
Most Part C plans cover
prescription drugs. You may
be able to add drug
coverage to some plan
types. If not already
included.

Chapter 4
Decoding Medicare Part D for your Prescriptions

Medicare Part D can seem like being on a Roller coaster. Understanding and controlling your prescription costs is key. We're going to delve deeply into the realm of prescription drug plans. So, make sure your harness is on, my friend. This knowledge will empower you to use this tool like an expert and get you some control over your healthcare decisions.

To begin with, why should you give part D any thought at all? Consider this: With health and happiness in hand, you're enjoying your retirement when – bam! – the cost of prescription drugs can be rather burdensome. If we live long enough odds are we'll need some sort of prescription drugs.

Part D comes into play here. It's your financial defense against skyrocketing expense of prescription drugs; it is more than just a feature of Medicare. You're swimming with sharks and no cage if you don't have it. There could also be penalties if you don't enroll when you are first eligible.

Comprehending the Blueprint. Part D is like a puzzle, and each piece represents a different aspect of your prescription drug coverage. Here's what you'll need to comprehend to put it all together:

Timing is crucial for enrollment, just as much as the coverage itself. You have deadlines to meet and windows to watch. Enroll as soon as possible during the initial Enrollment Period or when you discontinue another reputable plan to incur late enrollment penalties that linger longer than a cold or covid.

Late Enrollment Penalty for Part D

Selecting A Plan: Not every Part D plan is made equally. Every plan includes a formulary or list of approved medications specifying which drugs are covered and how much you must pay. Consider it like selecting the appropriate fishing bait as an example. The right bait or lure will land you a whale, while the incorrect one will only leave you with old tires and boots.

The costs associated with prescription drugs are comprised of four main components: premiums, deductibles, copayments, and coinsurance. Comprehending these terms is essential to avoid overspending on necessary medications as each plan applies a different price tag.

The Gap in Coverage: the famous donut hole will be gone in 2025. However, there is still a possible $2000 out of pocket. This coverage gap may ambush you like a robber in the night. This wouldn't be ideal – especially if you were ill or trying to cover – having large, unexpected bills could make you sick.

I take it you are aware of the Inflation Reduction Act. If you are new to Medicare. I suspect you're not. You may have seen some headlines or heard people complaining about increases or having to change plans.

Of course, advertising will be putting a spin on savings – not telling you how things are going to be sliced up. Insurance companies aren't going to just reduce out of pocket and absorb the cost.

What they are not going to tell you is this:

Max Out of Pocket "MOOP" with a $2000 cap

That's right, there will be a cap on the amount of money you spend out of pocket for prescriptions. The dreaded Donut Hole is gone in 2025.

The amount is set at $2,000. However, let's be real before you exhale with relief. This will help if you're struggling with expensive meds. How is it going to be for you? Where is the cost going to be shifted?

$35 Monthly Cap on Insulin

 This is a big one too. If you rely on insulin, 2025 is the year you stop paying through the nose for it. You'll only have to pay $35 a month – which will be a blessing for a lot of people. What are the ripples? What about other meds? What about the cost of the plan? Will it be increased?

Gaining control of this Game

Now how do you master this game? Here's your strategy:

Review Annually: Plans change, prices adjust, and your needs evolve. Review your plans each year during the Open Enrollment Period. It's like Checking your nets for holes; necessary maintenance to ensure the best catch. I, of course, recommend consulting your agent – they'll likely be up to date with the changes and options. Why mess around?

Manage medications: work with your doctor to see if there are more cost-effective alternatives for your prescriptions like generic options or can you make diet and lifestyle changes? Would it make sense to check on getting a methylation test to see if you're deficient in anything or how your body processes vitamins and minerals. You might just need supplementation?

Get Extra Help: If your wallet is thinner than a dieting cat or dog and you're struggling to make ends meet, you may be eligible for Extra Help, a program designed to help low-income people with their prescription expenditures.

Remain Up to Date: Keep an eye out for new possibilities, read the fine print, and comprehend the changes. The compass that helps you navigate the confusing waters of Medicare Part D is information. Check our social media and newsletters for changes and inside info.

Concluding Remarks: Part D is more than simply a section in your Medicare handbook. It's a lifesaver that prevents the weight of prescription expenses from capsizing your retirement vessel. This component of Medicare can become a valuable tool in your health management arsenal if you know what to look for and take a strategic approach.

Here you have it: the insider information on Medicare Part D, intended to protect you from any hazards associated with managing your healthcare in retirement, as well as enlighten you. Recall that having knowledge about Medicare is not only advantageous but also essential. Stay sharp, stay savvy, and let part D work for you not against you. Welcome to smarter healthcare management, and goodbye to prescription worries!

Chapter 5
Medicare Supplement Plans (Medigap) Cracking the Code on Extra Coverage

Welcome to the secret Vault of Medicare – the world of Medigap or Med Supps.

This isn't about splurging on extras; this is about protecting yourself from the barrage of unforeseen medical expenditures that Medicare allows to fall between the gaps.

Many go what we call" going naked" or in MN – "going out in the cold without a coat"– which basically means not having additional coverage and depending only on original Medicare (Parts A and B). Using this method may expose you to large out of pocket costs. Your hospital and medical expenses are mostly covered by original Medicare, but not entirely.

Deductibles, copayments, and coinsurance are examples of critical gaps. For example, although Part A pays for hospital stays in general, it has a large deductible per benefit period and does not pay for stays in skilled care facilities or hospitals that are longer than a predetermined amount of time.

Part B pays for 80% of authorized medical care, the other 20% is your responsibility with no cap on out-of-pocket expenses. This can be very expensive for major illnesses or lengthy treatments. This could be an expensive ordeal without a supplement plan

What a Medicare Supplement Policy Covers:

The following expenses are usually or fully covered by a Medicare Supplement Policy.

1. Part A Deductible: Part A is the amount you have to pay before Medicare Begins to pay for hospital expenses. Medicare Supplement policies can cover this amount.

2. Part A Coinsurance: For inpatient stays, this covers hospital expenses beyond the deductible.

3. Part B Coinsurance: The 20% coinsurance that you would typically have to pay for part B services is covered by a Medicare supplement.

4. Part A Hospice Care Coinsurance: Medicare Supplements might take over and pay the coinsurance if you require hospice care.

5. Coinsurance for Skilled Nursing Facility (SNF) Care: After the initial coverage term, a Medicare supplement might assist with the coinsurance for skilled nursing facility care.

6. Part B Excess Charges: Medicare Supplements will pay the difference if your healthcare provider bills you more than Medicare has approved.

Picking the best Medicare Supplement Policy:

Medicare supplements provide many letter designated standardized plans, Such as Plan A, Plan F, and Plan G. Insurance companies do not differ in the coverage provided by the plans, nevertheless, the rates may vary, and there is MA, MN, and WI with their unique plans.

Choosing the right plan depends on your specific needs and budget. Some plans offer comprehensive coverage, while others offer plans covering specific gaps. To make an informed choice, you must evaluate your financial status and healthcare needs.

Signing up for Medicare Supplements:

The best time to enroll is during your Medicare Supplement Open Enrollment Period. This period starts when you're 65 or older and enrolled in Part B. Insurance companies are not allowed to refuse you coverage or raise your premiums during this time due to your health.

Many like a Medicare supplement plan as it provides more options. Basically, you can use it anywhere Medicare is accepted – which is just about everywhere. It generally costs more. However, each person's needs are unique and depending on budget, health, location, and other factors one plan whether it's a

Medicare supplement combined with a Part D drug plan or a Medicare Advantage plan that includes drugs should all be considered.

Many like to think of a supplement plan a "pay before you need it" and an advantage plan as a "pay if you need to use it." All options should be considered.

Medicare Supplement vs. Medicare Advantage:

It's crucial to understand you can't have a Medicare Advantage plan and a Medicare Supplement at the same time. Depending on your needs and tastes, you'll have to select one or the other. Many think of a Medicare Supplement plan as pay before you need it and Medicare Advantage after and if you need it. They both have pluses and minuses. We'll cover these as we go.

Staying informed is Key:

You'll want to understand the complexities and review your policies each year to make sure you have the right coverage in place. These plans can provide peace of mind, especially when unexpected healthcare costs arise.

We'll discuss Medicare Enrollment periods and the significance of making educated decisions during them in our next chapter.

Chapter 6
Enrollment Periods (AEP) (GEP) (IEP) (OEP) (SEP)
What the Heck is the Big Deal?

Alrighty then, Listen up. These are important dates, and if you're reading this, you're probably really trying to figure it out. Don't worry. This is completely normal and you're not alone. I'm hoping this book helps. I had to read a lot of them to get a grasp.

But don't worry. Stay with me – we're going to get through this together.

Enrolling in Medicare isn't the one size that fits all or do it when you get around to it affair. I know what you're thinking and agree – it shouldn't be this difficult!

What People Get Wrong (And How You Can Avoid Being Locked Out)

Just thinking about the last couple of weeks and cases we had…

I had a person – we'll call him Harold - just take original Medicare Parts A with no Part B or Part D. I see it all the time. Harold and people like him are confused and become paralyzed by all the options. They don't go to the doctor anyway. So, they put it off - don't do anything and hope for the best. It's frustrating when they finally call but it's totally understandable how it happens.

This is very risky – especially if one doesn't have a lot of money to cover the gaps. 20% of medical bills can be a load. I'm still trying to help him.

I had another guy – we'll call him uncle "Cheapskate Charlie" not take part B or Part D when he was first eligible. He has penalties and doesn't qualify for special exceptions.

- Medicare Part B Penalty: is 10% of part B premium for every 12-month period that they could have had part B but didn't sign up. The worst part is it lasts forever. That's what the heck!

- Medicare Part D (Prescription Drug Coverage) Penalty: If there isn't from an employer or union – the penalty is calculated by 1% by the number of months he went without coverage.

For example, if someone goes without Part D for 12 months, the penalty would be 12% added to the monthly part D premium.

I heard all about this mess after Cheapskate Charlie called when his wife was in the hospital and asked about getting health insurance for her. He was waiting for her to turn 65. She didn't have coverage from his employer's plan after he retired and started Medicare. Aye! What the Heck indeed!

These are the key enrollment periods:

1. Initial Enrollment Period (IEP) This is your first opportunity to enroll in Medicare, and it spans seven months. Three months before your 65th birthday, your birthday month, and three months after. It's best not to miss this window or double check with a pro – not the neighbor, not with know-it-all Barb from work who retired last year and moved to Florida or Uncle Cheapskate, to make sure you can wait.

   If you have creditable coverage from an employer or spouses' coverage you may not need it. If not, delayed coverage and penalties are probable.

2. General Enrollment Period (GEP): If you missed your IEP or didn't sign up for Part B when you were first eligible, you can enroll during GEP, it takes place every year from January 1st to March 31st, each year. However, you can be

charged for late enrollment, and your coverage won't begin until July 1ˢᵗ

3. Special Enrolment Periods (SEP): If you meet specific requirements. SEPs allow you to enroll in Medicare outside of the regular enrollment periods. These include things like retiring after 65 or having your employer's insurance terminated.

4. Annual Enrollment Period (AEP). It takes place from October 15th to December 7th. You'll know as there will be a ton of advertising targeting you. You can switch plans, adjust Part D or switch to Medicare advantage from original Medicare and make other adjustments.

This is a busy time of year so it's best to mark your calendar and put a reminder to schedule a review if needed as they could be difficult to obtain. It's estimated over 11,000 people a day are turning 65 and with recent changes those with plans already are reviewing to make sure they are good.

Here's the deal: Every year, plans can change. What worked for you last year might not work this year. Maybe you moved into an area that has a 5-star Medicare advantage plan and the clinic is a couple of blocks away. Maybe the drug you need isn't covered.

Don't mess around. The Annual Enrollment Period, or AEP as we call it, is your opportunity to review and if needed make changes. Being in the insurance business for about 20 years I've learned to never assume anything. You shouldn't either. Find a good local expert agent. They should know what's available in your area and give you some options. It doesn't cost anything more to use an agent, an experienced agent or no agent. It's all the same.

Remember what works for one person may not be the best choice or option for another. Plans and networks can be different – even in the same state. Don't assume one company or plan that is recommended by someone other - than an insurance expert - is a good plan for you.

 In our next Chapter, we'll debunk some more Medicare myths and misconceptions to make sure you have accurate information or know where to look.

Chapter 7
Common Medicare Myths Debunked

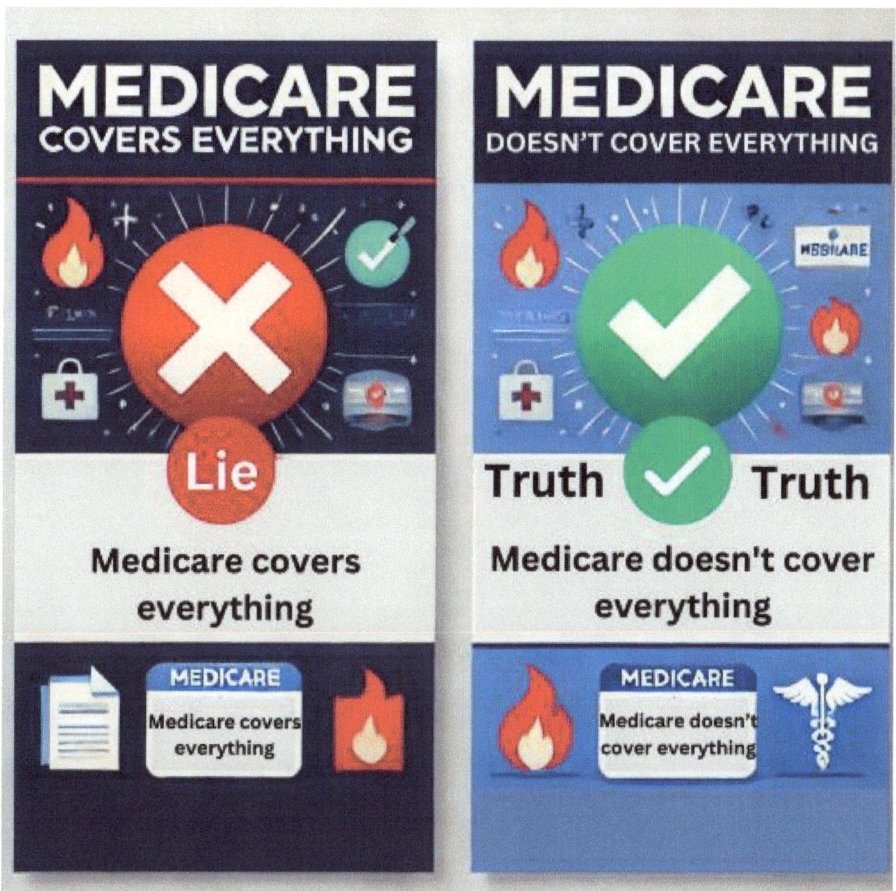

Our mission and we've chosen to accept it is to ensure you have the most accurate and up to date Medicare information. We're clearing up some of those common misconceptions about Medicare in this chapter

Myth 1: Medicare Covers Everything

This is probably the most common myth about Medicare. To be honest – I thought when I turned 65, (I'm not 65 yet) Health care would no longer be something to worry about. You probably were thinking the same thing?

While Medicare can offer great coverage, it doesn't cover everything. There are gaps in coverage. There is no or little coverage for dental, vision, hearing, and long-term care. That is where Medicare Supplement or Medicare Advantage plans come into play.

Myth 2: Medicare Doesn't cost anything

For most people who have worked and paid into Medicare for at least ten years, Part A is free. Part B has charges and other supplemental coverage have charges too. To make sure you get the coverage you need, you must budget for these rates.

Myth 3: Medicare and Medicaid are the same thing

These are two different programs. Medicare and Medicaid. Medicare is mostly for those age 65 or older. Conversely, Medicaid is a combined federal and state program that offers low-income individuals and families access to healthcare coverage.

Myth 4: You Get Automatically Enrolled in Medicare

While some people are automatically enrolled when they turn 65, it's not the case for everyone. If you're not getting social security at 65 you'll need to enroll.

Myth 5: You Can't Change Plans

You can make changes during Annual Enrollment Period (AEP). The AEP gives you the chance to make changes, such as moving from Original Medicare to an Advantage plan, changing your Part D prescription drug coverage, or doing other things.

Myth 6: Medicare Covers You in Other Countries

With a few exceptions, such as emergencies, Original Medicare usually doesn't cover medical services outside of the U.S.A. However, there are some advantage plans that offer international coverage if you're a traveler.

Myth 7: You can't get Medicare if you are still working

If you have employer sponsored health insurance and are still employed, you can still get Medicare. Sometimes, the employer plan is a better option. It's up to you to decide if you should enroll in Part B. You will want to check with your Human Resources Department to check and see what is available.

Myth 8: All Medicare Plans Are the same

Medicare advantage plans. Part D prescription drug plans and Medicare Supplement policies can vary significantly as far as cost, coverage, and networks. It's imperative to compare plans to find the one that best aligns with your needs.

Hopefully, we've debunked some of these common myths. Our goal is to make you aware and provide clarity so you can make the right choices and not have major setbacks or surprises while you're retired.

In the next chapter, we'll explore financial aspects of Medicare, including costs, premiums, and ways to manage expenses. So, keep going!

Chapter 8
Managing the Costs and Expenses of Medicare

In this chapter, we cover various costs associated with Medicare and explore ways to manage costs.

Unfortunately, Medicare isn't free, although it does provide a lot of services. Depending on your budget, needs and risk tolerance, some plans and options will make more sense than others.

1. Part A Premium For most Medicare Part A (hospital insurance) recipients don't pay a premium, some may if they haven't worked and and have paid Medicare taxes for a minimum of ten years. Because the premium might add up, it's important to account for it in your budget.

2. Part B Premium: The monthly premium for Part B (medical insurance) is subject to change based on your income. To keep your Part B, you must pay this payment to maintain coverage.

3. Part B Deductible: Before Part B coverage begins, you must pay a deductible each year. Be ready to pay for this upfront.

4. Part B Coinsurance and Copayments: For most of the part B services, you will normally be required to pay 20% of the Medicare approved amount. This covers medical supplies, outpatient care, and appointments with doctors.

5. Part D Premium: You will have to pay a monthly premium if you decide to sign up for a Part D prescription drug plan. Plan rates can differ, so compare options to find the best deal.

6. Part D deductible and Drug Costs: Part D plans may have various drug cost categories and deductibles. Budgeting for your prescription drugs might be easier if you are aware of these expenses.

7. Medicare Supplement "Medigap" Premium: If you have a Medicare supplement policy, you'll pay a separate premium to the insurance company. The Amount can vary depending on the plan. The most common seems to be Plan G or the Extended basic plan in MN as they fill most of the gaps. The average premium for a supplement is around $130 - $250 a month.

Managing healthcare expenses:

You'll want to come up with some tactics to make sure you can afford any medical bills in retirement.

1. Set a Budget: Established health care budget that takes out of pocket expenses, deductibles, and premiums into consideration. You can make better plans if you are aware of your financial obligations.

2. There may be Low Income Assistance available: You might be eligible for Medicaid or Extra Help, which can help with Medicare expenses if your income is and resources are ow.

3. Compare Plans Every year: Examine your Medicare plan choices at the Annual Enrollment Period. (AEP). The short cut is to use an experienced local agent as they will likely be on top of all the changes and plans in your area. It doesn't cost anything to use an experienced local agent.

4. Make Use of preventive procedures: Medicare offers preventive procedures that are frequently free. Maintaining your health can help cut costs in the future and of course live better.

5. Examine Your Needs for Prescription Drugs: If you have prescription drugs research if there is a way to get off them or natural ways to address issues. Review your Part D plan annually too.

6. Consider Medicare Advantage and Supplement plans. If you just have Original Medicare, you could be exposed to large co-pays. Some Medicare Advantage Plans are free. For some their Doctors and Networks could work well in the area. Is there a five-star plan in your area?

In your retirement years, keep in mind that proactive healthcare cost management can result in financial peace of mind. The last thing you want to worry about is having a ton of medical bills. Do be afraid to consult with Medicare experts.

Mastering Medicare: Strategies for Unlocking Healthcare after 65.

You are no doubt surprised Medicare isn't as easy as you thought it would be. I know. I thought it'd be one less thing to worry about. It can be.

I hope you found some help in this book. Medicare is not a one size fits all program. Every person has different demands and needs which are influenced by things like age, health, preferred doctors, financial situation, network accessibility, and even one's zip code. What is Ideal for one person may not be the best choice for you.

You know, I've been there... as mentioned I've read countless books on Medicare, trying to make sense of it all, and let me tell you—sometimes it felt like I was getting further from understanding, not closer! Even at the carrier meetings - I noticed there weren't many agents who seemed like they were experts. When that one author even said, "The more I studied Medicare, the less I knew." I mean, Aye! What a mess, right? Hopefully, this has helped. You'll get there. If you have questions or need help reachout.

A carrier rep told me to look at a Medicare supplement "Medigap" plan as a pay before you go and a Medicare advantage as a pay when you go. It helped me for some reason. Start there. If you're super healthy don't use much healthcare and maybe have some HSA money saved up – then look at some Advantage plans. Most are low or even zero cost. if you have a lot of health issues and need some surgeries – then look at supplement plans. There is more to it but start there. There are almost always better options than just going naked with original Medicare. Which one is best for you?

I'm here to provide you with some crucial advice on how to use Medicare effectively, maximize your coverage, and make sure your medical requirements are satisfied.

Stay up to Date:

Stay informed about enrollment periods, coverage revisions, and modifications. Your greatest tool for making wise decisions is knowledge.

Subscribe to our **Facebook** page

https://www.facebook.com/**VitalShieldUSA**

https://www.instagram.com/tpeddyco/

and other social media. We have a newsletter, and you can always DM or email me.

VitalShield Insurance Services:

333 N Washington Ave Suite #300, Minneapolis, MN 55401

763.290.1267 https://vitalshieldus.com/

To Dawn,

I'm grateful for you! I don't know where I'd be if I hadn't met you. I appreciate you being the woman you are and never settling. You've been a solid foundation through every step from when we were teenagers and young parents until now. I truly landed on my feet with you in my life. Thank you for being my partner and rock.

To Pam

I appreciate your positive attitude and unwavering support. "You are in charge" Thank you for being here from day one as we built the agency with focus on health, life, and Medicare insurance. You're such a reliable, competent, and friendly presence in our agency, always taking care of our clients. Your hard work and commitment do not go unnoticed, and I deeply appreciate your continued support and enthusiasm.